A HANDBOOK OF

MEL'S TIPS

FOR

HEALTHY LIVING

EMPOWER | MOTIVATE

THE POWER OF
POSSIBILITIES

BY **MEL ZUCKERMAN**

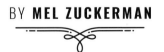

Published by the Canyon Ranch® Press
8600 East Rockcliff Road, Tucson, Arizona 85750 USA

Printed in the United States of America

Canyon Ranch® is a registered trademark of
CR License, LLC.

www.canyonranch.com

Design by CR Products, LLC
Teri Bingham and Christopher Sahlin

Library of Congress Control Number: 2017951974

MEL'S TIPS FOR HEALTHY LIVING
Zuckerman, Mel

ISBN 978-0-9624102-3-9

THIS BOOK IS DEDICATED TO

the memory my late father,
Norman Zuckerman,
a lifelong smoker who had many opportunities
to change, but spent his last months repeating
"If only I had …"

*It's of value to think of health as that condition of the
individual that makes possible the highest enjoyment of
life. Health, when thought of simply as the absence of
disease, is a standard of mediocrity, but when thought
of as a quality of life it is a standard of inspiration
and ever-increasing achievement.*

–Jesse F. Williams, M.D., circa 1930

contents

Foreword

by Richard Carmona, M.D., M.P.H., FACS,
17th Surgeon General of the United States (2002-2006)

In 1900, the average American could expect to live around 50 years and probably die of an infectious disease. A little more than a century later, life expectancy is approaching 80 years, and America's and the world's consciousness regarding health, wellness and prevention is on the rise. Every day we understand more about the relationships between our genes and our environment, and it is becoming increasingly clear that the environment we live in and the way we behave have profound effects, both positive and negative, on our genome. The behaviors we choose daily may overcome or reduce genetic predisposition to disease, or, conversely, increase risk or make illness worse. And it's worth noting that 2015 saw the first decline in decades, though slight, of U.S. life expectancy.

Almost 40 years ago, Enid and Mel Zuckerman had a vision that was ahead of its time, to create an inspirational environment where people could come to pursue optimal health and wellness, and appreciate life's endless possibilities. Immersed in a national system of "sick care," Canyon Ranch is a beacon of hope and a model for true health care that has continued to evolve to its present iconic stature. This is largely because of Mel's passion, persistence and vision. He continues to ignore his chronological clock to this day, truly embodying the principles of "living younger longer."

I have often said that something like the Canyon Ranch model—where health professionals are compensated for guiding people toward optimal health via prevention strategies—is what our nation needs to move forward in this arena. No strategy to transform the U.S. healthcare system can be complete or successful without aggressively incorporating the Canyon Ranch approach to prevention and healthy lifestyles. In fact, 75 cents of every one of the $3 trillion we spend on health care annually in this country goes to treating chronic diseases, most of which can be prevented or improved by lifestyle.

Mel walks the talk, and the course of his life shows the benefits of doing just that. His driving passion is to help all of us achieve optimal health and wellness in order to live younger longer. Between these book covers lies an authentic path to the Fountain of Youth. I hope you embrace the journey!

Richard Carmona

Richard Carmona, M.D., M.P.H., FACS
17th Surgeon General of the United States (2002-2006)
Chief of Health Innovations, Canyon Ranch

Introduction

I regularly give a talk I think of as "living younger longer" to our guests at Canyon Ranch. I usually do it early in the day, for a roomful of people who've mostly been up for an hour or two already, out walking and having a healthy breakfast.

I always start by telling them where I got the title of the talk. It's a play on words, based on something I heard the noted anthropologist Ashley Montagu say at a conference in 1982. He was explaining that we get the whole concept of fitness from the ancient Greeks, whose ideal, as Montagu put it, was "to die young ... as late as possible!" After a moment of reflection, most of the audience members understand and smile.

We can pull off the trick of dying young as late as possible because each of us has two clocks running throughout our lives. One is our chronological clock, determined by the date on our birth certificate, and we can't do a thing about that. Fortunately, we have a good deal of control over the second one, our biological clock, which measures our physiological and biological age, and determines how well we function. The ancient Greeks obviously meant that the best possible thing was "to die young" *biologically*, "as late as possible" *chronologically*. I interpret that thought as living younger longer, the theme of my talk and of this book.

A doctor can calculate your biological age by looking at a set of biomarkers that measure how old your body really is—things like aerobic capacity, how robust your immune system is, how much bone and muscle you have, how your body uses sugar, and so on. The good news is that over the past few decades, the medical community has discovered that virtually every one of those biomarkers is 70 to 80 percent reversible. In other words, while you can't turn back the hands on your chronological clock, you can reset your biological clock significantly. (By the way, I believe that there's another important clock ticking, your psychological clock—how old you think of yourself as being. As long as we feel well and energized, we all pretty much think of ourselves as 25.)

The bad news, as many people seem to see it, is that you are the only person who can do the work of rewinding the hands on your biological clock. That is, you can't pop a magic pill that will roll back the years as you sleep, and you can't pay someone to make you biologically younger while you finish a bag of chips on the couch. You are the best doctor you will ever have. And quite simply, the best treatment you can prescribe for yourself is to adopt a healthy lifestyle and stick with it. If you do, your quality of life will be vastly improved.

"Quality of life" is an elusive phrase that has a different meaning for each of us. So my goal is to inspire you to think clearly about what that means to you, and I give you many ways to reach that goal by following the practices in this book regularly.

Imagine yourself 10, 20, even 40 years from now. What would you like to be doing? Will you be able to walk around the lake? Work in your garden? Play tennis or ski? Start a second career? If you want that future, now's the time to prepare.

For the first 50 years of my life, I lived with lots of physical limitations. I abdicated everything in regard to my health, well-being and aging to my doctors, to drugs and to fate. I still believe in fate, but I also believe that there is a lot you can do about fate, if you choose. Look at me for a real-life example. Before my *Aha!* moment at age 50, I could not have imagined a future where I'd ever be able to walk a mile and a half, much less jog it in a time that put me in the top end of my age class. But with the help of a great trainer, I achieved it after just 10 days of walking and jogging. When I realized what I had done, my life changed forever.

Whether you see yourself climbing Everest at 60, keeping up with your children or grandchildren, or just radiating energy and vitality in your everyday activities when you take charge of the quality of your life by making it a priority, you'll enjoy a higher level of health, wellness and hope. And the equation works both ways: The more you improve your level of health and wellness, the more likely you are to see the quality of your life rising—no matter how old you are.

You don't need me to tell you that the arrow of time goes only one way, or to remind you that aging is not a great process. There's a growing chorus of people out there complaining about getting old and bemoaning the loss of physical functionality and increasing cognitive impairment that usually begins in our 60s and gets worse from that point on. Aging has become a dirty word.

So why *do* I offer this little book about health and highlight this nasty subject—aging? Well, partly it's because, I'm nearing 90, and I've done a lot of it. But mostly it's because for 40 or so years I've been an impassioned proponent of healthy living and a student of its effects on the aging process. In trying to communicate to Canyon Ranch guests the importance of living well every day, I have learned that change begins when we really take in the hard truth that the aging process begins the moment we are born. The human body peaks between 25 and 35, and for some athletes, even younger than that. So in reality, we're all going downhill after young adulthood.

That may sound grim, but what I want you to realize is this: Even though you can't alter the direction of the journey, you can have an enormous impact on its quality. If, starting today, you decide to reset your biological clock and make lifestyle choices that raise your level of wellness, you will immediately feel better, and you'll be redrawing your map of the possibilities ahead. In fact, the major payoffs of your decision could be 10, 20, 30 or even 40 years ahead of you. Trust me, those years pass quickly and you will reap what you sow.

The healthy lifestyle I adopted decades ago has given me more than I ever could have hoped for or imagined. The sickly, overweight, anxious individual I was in middle age—the guy whose battery of tests once showed, at age 40, that he had the biomarkers of a 65- to 70-year-old—has actually gotten to live to a good age. When I turned 65, I underwent a much more sophisticated set of tests to once again determine my biological age: They showed that at that time I had the body of a 45- to 50-year old. So, while living through 25 busy, productive years in real time, my healthy lifestyle whittled them right off my biological age.

I'm in active retirement, still enjoying life, at nearly 90. In the past few years, I've had the joy of watching our family's wonderful "baby surge"—with grandchildren and great-grandchildren. Would I have been here to see them, to hold them in my arms, if I hadn't "cleaned up my act"? I'm virtually certain that I would have been just a few stories and a picture on the wall to these children.

There are many payoffs for healthy living, but this is probably the ultimate one: You get to see the future.

This is not a textbook on lifestyle, health and wellness. I imagine you've had access to many of those, whether you've read them or not. Nor is this book meant to vastly improve your IQ on these subjects. It is meant more to address your EQ (emotional quotient), because in order to step toward real change, you need to access every emotional asset you have. Readiness. Intention. Commitment. Discipline. These are the inner resources that will see you through the process of embracing a healthy lifestyle and let you enjoy all its present and long-term benefits. If you aren't interested in developing those qualities, then my advice to you is to stop reading now. (The only part of the book you would probably feel comfortable with is "To Hell With Health: The Definitive Pocket Guide to Getting Older Faster," which illuminates a certain kind of willful self-deception about health habits—a type of thinking that a surprising number of people choose to engage in. You'll find it between Chapters 6 and 7.)

So, are you committed enough to live to be part of your grandchildren's lives? Disciplined enough to reach a vital, vigorous old age? Ready to tap the reserves of energy and resilience you haven't seen since you were a kid? Good. Keep your eye on the life you'd most like to have in the years ahead. Set an intention to move toward it every day. Then take one step. And another.

Don't be overwhelmed—this handbook is a compilation of rules, principles and practices for healthy living, boiled down and made as simple as possible. It's the very best of what I've learned living at Canyon Ranch for four decades, surrounded by experts in every field related to health. The basics aren't up for discussion: You must exercise. You must eat a good diet the majority of the time. You must keep your weight at a reasonable level, get a good night's sleep, manage stress and, above all, you must not smoke. You must also stay closely connected to others and have purpose in life. But how you do that is up to you, and what follows is a collection of different ways to think about these nonnegotiable rules for a healthy, fulfilling life—ways that have worked for thousands of guests of Canyon Ranch— and dozens of tips for implementing them. My hope is that they help you live the life you want.

Some of the practices and tips you find here may already be favorites of yours. Others will strike you as good ideas and that might work for you. Some won't. No one could do everything in this book at once—that would be crazy! So, in every chapter, pick a few things and try them. Mix it up. Surprise yourself. And use that intention, commitment and discipline of yours to find out just what would happen if you stuck to a few potential new habits—even just one—for a month. If you're looking for inspiration, or a boost to stay on track, you'll find it in these pages.

One thing you'll notice: Regular exercise shows up, in some fashion, in most every chapter. If there's one universal game-changer, that's it. If you do nothing else, skim for the one fact, suggestion or tidbit that inspires you to move your body. Then do it.

There is one health truism that no scientific research has ever contradicted in all these years: It is easier to preserve health than to repair it. The path to optimal health is clearly defined—walking it is still up to you.

Read on or close the book. Whatever you choose, I wish you the best on your journey of life.

chapter **1**
WHAT YOU NEED TO MAKE LASTING CHANGES

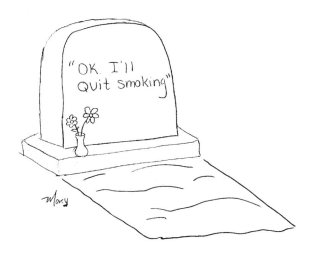

Giving up a habit—including the habit of sedentary living—is hard. But some people, the successful ones, manage to bridge the gap between what they know they should do and what they do. What enables them to make the leap? And how can I help them do that? These are questions that have been going around in my head for nearly 40 years.

For me, the feeling I got when I was released from the cage of not exercising was all I needed. I had severe asthma as a kid, and when I was just 8 years old, a doctor imposed a health myth on me and my parents: "Exercising will make his asthma worse," he told my already protective mom and dad. "If he exercises, he will become ill." With that, I was consigned to a life on the sidelines. But running for the first time at 50 liberated me, and in short order I was hooked.

Sadly, though, the wonderful feeling of moving just isn't enough for most people. They may have played hard in childhood, or taken up a sport in school, but now, they insist, they're busy. Work, family, commuting, obligations—there's no time for exercise. So they move less and less the older they get. They lose touch with the joy of it and leave exercise benched on the "someday I'll get around to it" list.

One answer to bridging the gap between "someday" and "now" is visiting Canyon Ranch. Enid and I built it expressly to give people an environment in which they could discover for themselves how good healthy living *feels*.

But even Canyon Ranch doesn't work for every guest and, of course, not everyone can spend time with us.

So the question remains pressing: What do people need to change their ways? What do you need?

The key is emotional energy. *You must consciously desire and value health as it should be valued*: as the irreplaceable foundation for everything else you love and enjoy to become responsible for your own health, well-being and aging process.

Obviously, health as measured by lack of illness can never be a promise. But scientific research shows you can improve your odds significantly. You can make practical, positive choices that enhance the quality of your daily life through the years—that is one measure of health that does come with a promise. It all starts when you set an intention to become responsible for your own health, well-being and aging process.

Health is a precious and positive thing over which we have a great deal of control. But far too many individuals don't realize that, not on a gut level. For them, the critical experience of emotional connection that I like to call the *Aha!* moment comes too late—as it did long ago for my father. He knew for years that he should stop smoking, but couldn't do it until his doctor told him he had lung cancer.

That's when the "Aha!"s usually occur: in a doctor's office, or in an emergency room or a cardiac care unit. And for too many people, the life-changing moment when they emotionally "get" the connection between their actions and their state of health is exceedingly painful. "If only I had … "—these are agonizing words to hear spoken in despair by someone you love. My father repeated them many times during the last months of his life, and they were devastating for both of us. This book is just my latest attempt to spare as many people as possible from having to endure that pain.

So what do you need to improve the way you live? Recent studies on successful habit change have produced a set of ideas known as the Self-Determination Theory.[1] Researchers in this field have identified three things we humans need to change for good:

FIRST, WE NEED AUTONOMY

the sense that we are making our own decisions for our own reasons.

THE SECOND FACTOR IS COMPETENCE

the conviction that we have the ability to change and can find help if we need it.

THE THIRD FACTOR IS RELATEDNESS

a personal connection with someone who cares and supports the change we are trying to make.

Perhaps this little book will help you with those three requirements—that's certainly my hope in writing it. I want to inspire you to make an autonomous decision—a decision from the bottom of your heart to live a healthier life. Here's a first step: Have an honest, introspective

---

[1]"Facilitating health behaviour change and its maintenance: Interventions based on Self-Determination Theory," by Richard M. Ryan, et al., *The European Health Psychologist*, Vol 10., March 2008.

conversation with yourself. Is your emotional self really ready for change? It's okay if the answer is no (or not yet!). If it's yes, though, move on to the next chapter in this book. It lists 25 compelling reasons to exercise. Whether you are motivated by the promise of a better sex life or a sharper mind, identify the ones that speak to you. Circle them if you like. Write in your own reasons too. Then when the morning comes (and it will) when you're asking yourself, "Why am I doing this again?" let those items remind you.

You'll find all the competence you could possibly need within these pages—the Canyon Ranch experts and information and strategies to get you started and keep you going. Create a customized plan for yourself by focusing on the items that will make the most difference in your life. You *know* what to do. So use the nuggets in this book to remind you and check yourself against. Have you slipped? Forgotten the bit about eating brightly colored vegetables or taking care of your snoring? OK, now you know. Now you can get back on course.

As for relatedness and support, maybe my voice in your head will help a bit, but you may need to find a physician or a qualified trainer, or maybe just join forces with an encouraging friend or spouse who can help keep you going. There are lots of resources and communities online for people who track things such as workouts and weight loss, and these virtual connections can be a great help.

*See the Resources list on page 111. It includes books, websites and other materials that you may find helpful.

Whatever resources you need to become active, eat well and give up any destructive habits you may have, I urge you to go out and find them.* I promise that you will be glad you did.

chapter **2**
WHY YOU NEED TO EXERCISE

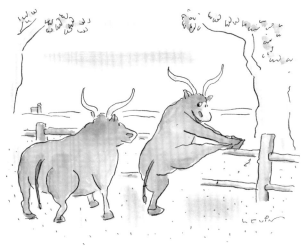

"I'm thinking of doing Pamplona this year."

2

You don't have to be an athlete—or a bull—to benefit from exercise.

Your body was built to move, and you *must* move it to be healthy. This is the hardest thing to get through to people. They'll go on crazy diets, spend fortunes on miracle cures and undergo surgeries and medical interventions. But they're incredibly resistant to hearing that the most important thing that they can possibly do for their health is to move their bodies! This drives me absolutely nuts, probably because I'd give anything if I could reach back and get my younger self into some jogging shoes.

So throughout this book, you will find me strongly emphasizing the benefits of exercise. I harp on it because it is so vital: Exercise, as my late friend Dr. Robert Butler once told the Senate Committee on Aging, is the only genuine Fountain of Youth. People have been seeking the fountain's magic since at least 1513, when Ponce de León took on the quest and discovered Florida instead. Now that we know the seemingly elusive secret is right under all of our noses, it seems crazy not to take advantage of it. It turned my life around, and I'm confident that it will do the same for you.

You don't have to take my word for it, though. I recommend a short video called, *23½ Hours: What Is the Single Best Thing We Can Do for Our Health?* by Dr. Mike Evans. It's an eye-opener and a potential lifesaver. Now take a look at this list, which pulls the highlights from the ever-growing mountain of research that documents exactly what you'll get from that "miracle cure" called exercise. Read on. And then get moving.

EXERCISE REDUCES CANCER RISKS.

The incidence or recurrence of cancer can be inhibited by exercise, according to some studies. Scientists have yet to determine if this is because of improved immune function, decreased stress or other factors.

EXERCISE PREVENTS OR SLOWS HEART DISEASE.

An active lifestyle reduces your chances of developing heart disease by nearly half. Why does that matter so much? More Americans die of heart disease every year than of any other cause.

EXERCISE PREVENTS THE ONSET OF TYPE-2 DIABETES.

The risk for developing diabetes—which leads to heart disease, nerve damage, vision loss, vascular disease, kidney failure and stroke—increases with age, except among very active people: Research on master endurance athletes in their 60s revealed that they had the same insulin and glucose profiles as young athletes. This suggests that diabetes is a disease of inactivity, not of age itself.

EXERCISE IS 50 PERCENT OF THE MOST EFFECTIVE TREATMENT FOR DIABETES.

The other half is a good diet. Regular exercise is powerful in treating diabetes because it improves insulin sensitivity for 24 to 36 hours. This means that if you exercise every day, your sensitivity to insulin will stay high, and your blood sugar will be better regulated naturally.

EXERCISE CLEARS EXCESS GLUCOSE FROM THE BLOOD.

During exercise, your muscles use sugar without needing insulin.

EXERCISING IS LIKE TAKING HEAVY-DUTY ANTIOXIDANTS.

Much like cars, our bodies can "rust out" over time as tissues are degraded by free radicals. (Unlike automobiles, however, our bodies have absolutely no trade-in value!) Exercise slows and even reverses the aging process by reducing inflammation, which is associated with most chronic disease processes, and releasing the body's own antioxidants.

EXERCISE RELIEVES STRESS THROUGH SHEER PHYSICAL RELEASE.

When something triggers the body's fight-or-flight reaction but there's no corresponding physical release (like fighting or running away), the result is stress. Physical exercise relaxes the body, gives the mind a rest and dependably lifts the spirits.

EXERCISE INCREASES MUSCLE MASS.

Greater muscle mass increases metabolism and improves the ratio of "good" to "bad" cholesterol in the blood. Muscle burns extra calories, even at rest.

EXERCISE STRENGTHENS THE BODY.

Strength-training exercise helps prevent gradual loss of bone and muscle with advancing age—a process that starts in the third decade of life and increases rapidly with age in sedentary people.

EXERCISE BURNS CALORIES.

That means you can eat more delicious, nutritious food and not put on fat.

EXERCISE HELPS YOU CONTROL YOUR WEIGHT.

In fact, for most people, maintaining a healthy weight is just about impossible without exercise.

EXERCISE KEEPS YOU YOUNGER AT A CELLULAR LEVEL.

The telomeres (or "handles") on the ends of the DNA strands of regular exercisers are on average as long as those of sedentary people who are 10 years younger. This is significant because shortening of telomeres appears to be one of the fundamental processes of aging. Yes, exercise even keeps your *cells* younger.

EXERCISE IMPROVES IMMUNE FUNCTION, SO YOU CATCH FEWER BUGS.

It does this in part by promoting efficient circulation of the lymph, the fluid that clears infection and toxins from the body.

EXERCISE MAKES YOU SMARTER.

It stimulates production of chemical messengers that function like fertilizer for brain cells. And studies have shown that people learn faster and remember better after a session of brisk exercise.

EXERCISE MAY HELP PROTECT YOU FROM DEVELOPING ALZHEIMER'S.

Research results are mixed on this, but most physicians advise patients who are concerned about dementia to exercise regularly.

EXERCISE MAKES YOU HAPPIER.

A 2010 study conducted using iPhones to survey people randomly about what they were doing and how happy they felt—a study that generated more than a quarter-million responses—found that exercise was the daily activity that made people second-happiest: People reported feeling happier when exercising than they did while conversing with friends, listening to music, eating, reading, etc. (I think you can guess which activity beat out even exercise on the happiness scale.)

EXERCISE IS AS EFFECTIVE AS ANTIDEPRESSANTS IN TREATING MILD TO MODERATE DEPRESSION.

Physical activity stimulates the release of soothing, mood-lifting chemicals into the bloodstream.

EXERCISE IMPROVES YOUR SEX LIFE.

In a study of overweight, sedentary men with erectile dysfunction, those who started exercising showed a significant improvement in sexual function. (Viagra and other such drugs work by increasing the body's sensitivity to nitric oxide, and exercise has been shown to increase levels of nitric oxide in the body.)

MANY FORMS OF EXERCISE GET YOU OUTSIDE.

There's no substitute for fresh air and time spent in the natural world. Studies confirm that outdoor exercise improves mood.

EXERCISE PROMOTES A GOOD NIGHT'S REST.

Regular exercise alone cures many cases of insomnia and poor sleep. (But not mine, unfortunately. I exercise for all the *other* reasons on this list.)

EXERCISE MAKES YOU LOOK BETTER.

What do you prefer? A beer gut or a fit, well-muscled, well-coordinated body? I'd say we all know which one looks younger and more attractive.

EXERCISE ALLOWS YOU TO RISE TO LIFE'S DEMANDS AND CHALLENGES.

When you're in good shape, you can play in the pool or go hiking or dancing or whatever else you feel like doing, whenever the opportunity arises. And you can change your own tire, carry your own groceries and lift your grandchildren.

EXERCISE MAKES YOU FEEL PROUD OF YOURSELF.

There's no more satisfying and legitimate source of self-esteem than knowing that you're taking good care of yourself.

EXERCISE IS FUN.

Ask any kid. And it can also be a great shared social activity.

FINALLY ...

Exercise relieves you of the need to make excuses for not exercising.

THE THREE PERCENT SOLUTION

How much would you pay for something that could deliver all the results on this list? How much would you pay if you could enjoy another year or two or five of great health?

I calculate that when all is said and done, if you devote just a measly three percent of your waking hours, approximately three to four hours a week, to maintaining your health, the long-term dividends—that bounty on the preceding list—will be remarkable. *Surely* you can invest that much time each week for your health and well-being. Remember that you get to do it your way, customizing your routine to your very particular preferences. That's what you'll begin to do in the next chapter.

Those who think they have not time for bodily exercise will sooner or later have to find time for illness.
— Edward Stanley, Earl of Derby (1826-93)

chapter **3**

HOW TO DEVELOP AN EXERCISE ROUTINE THAT WORKS FOR YOU

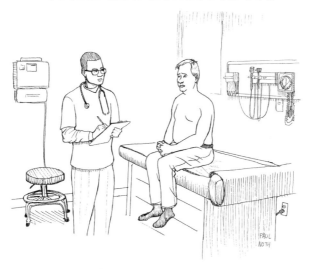

"Will I still be able to not exercise?"

"No," is the answer to that one. You've got to do it. So start with what you can make yourself do and gradually add more. If what you can do right now is walk slowly for 20 minutes, fine. Start there. Do it every day. As it gets easier—and it will—do more. (As a general rule, increase what you do by no more than 10 percent per week.)

Begin with just a small, achievable goal. Even one small step forward can make an enormous difference.

Aim for being a participant, not a perfectionist. Then you free yourself to try new things and to enjoy being a beginner. At Canyon Ranch, that's what we mean by the power of possibility.

Commit to working up a good sweat most days of the week. Optimally, shoot for at least 45 minutes of cardiovascular exercise four days a week, 15 to 20 minutes of strength training three nonconsecutive days a week, plus balance and agility work and stretching.

Everyone has the time to do this much. Remember: This is just three percent of your waking hours. I've heard possibly 1,000 people say they just don't have time to exercise, and I've never believed a single one of them. The real problem is never time. It's that they don't want to do it. And as long as they keep making excuses, they won't.

Sometimes, they've heard me describe what I do and almost unconsciously they feel they have to commit to *my* program, even though they're nothing like me. That, I can tell you with absolute confidence, is not going to work. There is no one-size-fits-all prescription. What works for someone else probably won't work for you. The trick is to find a routine that fits your circumstances and personality. The psychologists on our staff say that making that match is a pivotal step in making a lasting commitment. That's what this chapter will help you do: Get real about who you are and what will really work for you. Latch on to whatever feels like a fit and start building a routine from there.

One more key point: Even apart from working out, just try to sit less. Recent research focused solely on the amount of time people spent sitting still. It revealed that more than six hours of sitting a day significantly increased participants' chance of dying during the study. "Light, intermittent physical activity"—simply moving around—turns out to be vital to health. So take the stairs, get up and walk down the hall instead of using the phone, stroll to the coffee shop on your breaks, play with your kids on the living room floor. Let me say it again: **Just move.**

WHAT KIND OF EXERCISER ARE YOU?

The questions that follow will let you do some simple diagnostics of the "know thyself" variety. Take this self-knowledge seriously enough to apply it. What truly sounds like you? Focus there, and put together a plan that fits you like a favorite pair of broken-in jeans.

DO YOU FIND IT HARD TO GET GOING?

Basically, everybody does. The first few minutes are always the hardest, as your body changes physiological states from not moving to moving. So religiously follow the Five-Minute Rule: When you don't feel like exercising, suit up anyway and try it for just five minutes, that's all. If, after five minutes, you're too tired to continue, stop. You really do need rest. Nearly always, though, you'll be over the hump and keep going. Also, it really helps to warm up for five or 10 minutes with a slow, easy version of what you're going to do—walk for a while, then jog, before you run; swim a couple of easy laps before you go full on.

ARE YOU EASILY BORED?

Read on the elliptical machine or exercise bike. Listen to audio books. Exercise with a friend. If you need amusement, find it. And if you get bored with what you're doing, explore other forms of exercise. Have a different routine for each season of the year—swim in the summer and run on the treadmill in the winter, for instance. Polish up an old skill or learn something new. *What* you do is much less important than that you do *something* most days.

HAVE A LIMITATION OR PAIN THAT MAKES EXERCISE DIFFICULT?

Get into a pool. Moving in the water—the exercise you do can be as simple as just walking back and forth in a lap pool—has tremendous benefits, particularly for people with injuries, chronic illnesses or other limitations. Aquatic therapy is one of the first things hospitals have post-surgical patients do because it's so gentle, comfortable and safe. The overall resistance of the water helps strengthen the body in a balanced way, while the buoyancy, gentle enveloping pressure and the support provided by partial immersion offer unique advantages. If pain persists, of course, consider calling a professional for additional healing strategies.

Enid and I believe so much in the benefits of aquatic therapy for recovery from surgery and illness that we had a small pool built into our home. It's turned out to be invaluable. Plus, being in the water simply feels great.

LIKE GETTING YOUR MONEY'S WORTH?

Join a gym, club or yoga center. If getting value motivates you, you're likely to keep showing up. (But if you're not that sort of person, then don't waste your money.) Try different activities and classes to discover what you like and add variety and balance to your routine.

FUNCTION BEST WITH SOME STRUCTURE?

Hire a personal trainer or share one with a friend. Having an appointment to keep is very motivating, and a good trainer will help you ramp up your routine and keep it interesting. If you're a person who will always show up if you tell someone else you will, use that to your advantage and make a date.

DO YOU ENJOY ORGANIZED GROUP ACTIVITIES?

There are hundreds of exercise classes out there, from boot camp to dance to a dozen kinds of yoga. Try different activities and instructors, and change what you do whenever you feel like it. You may be surprised by what gives you a kick.

ARE YOU SOCIAL? LOVE DOING THINGS WITH FRIENDS?

Find a reliable workout buddy or join a group of walkers, hikers, joggers or swimmers. Once again, a commitment to someone else will help get you out the door, and you'll have fun. Health clubs and parks are great places to hang out and make friends. And if you don't like the atmosphere where you're working out, find another place. The world's full of gyms, parks and pools.

NEED TIME ALONE?

If your life is filled with work and family responsibilities, you may want to make your workout a time of quiet, a refuge from the demands of life. Running and swimming, in particular, are great activities for people who need to clear their heads.

MOTIVATED BY REWARDS?

Use that. Concentrate on how you'll reward yourself for working out with whatever you enjoy, whether it's a tasty (but not excessive) treat, an evening out or new workout clothes. You've earned it, so enjoy.

ARE YOU COMPETITIVE?

Well then, compete! Masters swim programs, orienteering meets, perimeter bicycle racing, triathlons, 5Ks and half-marathons, tennis and racquetball leagues and regular pickup soccer and basketball games are just a few of the possibilities for competitive types. And many of us find that the best competition, once we've come to enjoy the habit of exercise, is with ourselves. Set goals and measure your progress—it's powerfully motivating! Having said all that, I don't believe it's ultimately about competition. It's about keeping on keeping on. In my late 80s, I simply can't do what I once did. With age or any physical setbacks, you need to reset your goal. Just don't stop—readjust!

DREAM OF ADVENTURE?

The ambition to climb a mountain, hike a canyon or run a river can be a terrific motivator. Book the big trip and you'll have a definite reason to start a training program and stick with it.

LOVE KEEPING RECORDS AND TRACKING THINGS?

Buy yourself all the monitoring equipment you like: A computer for your bike, a heart-rate monitor, the latest wearable fitness trackers gauge your progress privately or online where you can compare your achievements with those of others. If you've got a little kid inside that loves gold stars, stick them on your calendar on days when you work out. Something that seems silly to someone else may help keep you on track. And how silly is that?

ENJOY BEING OUTSIDE?

Then don't try to make yourself go to the gym—hike, bike, walk, run in the great outdoors instead. Join an exercise group that meets outside, in a park.

I happen to live in ideal terrain for hiking, which is hands-down my favorite form of exercise. Over the years I've found both physical challenge and spiritual adventure on the trail—I feel at one with nature and at peace with myself while I'm hiking. I know that many Canyon Ranch guests experience something similar, because a number of them come just to hike, day after day. They've discovered that there's nothing better for body and soul.

RATHER STAY HOME?

Millions of people keep fit with television exercise programs, DVDs and active computer gaming systems. Or buy an exercise bike. I bet you can make room in your home for one favorite piece of cardio equipment. Maybe a bench and some free weights, too. It doesn't need to take much room or cost a fortune.

NEED ENCOURAGEMENT?

Open yourself to inspiration wherever you find it. Remember, it's all about self-determination. You've got to want to do it.

FOUR REALLY BAD EXCUSES FOR NOT WORKING OUT

1. I DIDN'T WORK OUT YESTERDAY (OR FOR THE LAST MONTH OR FOR THE LAST DECADE).

Yesterday doesn't matter. Only what you do today counts.

2. I'M IN BAD SHAPE.

Where you're at is irrelevant. The *direction of change* is what's important.

3. MY MUSCLES ARE SORE FROM YESTERDAY'S WORKOUT.

Mild-to-moderate muscle soreness is a sign that you're making progress. Working out again will make you feel better. So will mild analgesics, a massage or a warm bath with salts. Or all three.

If you're getting *very* sore, you're doing too much, too soon. Back off a little. But not all the way. (Joint soreness is another matter: Consult a physician, exercise physiologist or physical therapist for achy joints. And know that ice is your friend: Professional athletes are very consistent in icing problem joints.)

4. I DON'T LIKE THE WAY I LOOK IN MY WORKOUT CLOTHES, BATHING SUIT, ETC.

There's only one way to make yourself happier about your body, and that's to give it the activity it needs. Avoid looking in the mirror and keep your chin up— it'll get better.

If you worry that other people at the gym or pool are judging you—forget about it.

Everyone's obsessed with his or her own workout. If someone seems to notice you, don't take it personally— there's not much visual distraction on the treadmill or exercise bike, so people tend to focus on everyone who goes by out of sheer need for something new to look at. It's no big deal. And honestly, if you're still convinced that someone is judging you harshly, ask yourself, "What do I care what goes on in that person's mind?"

chapter 4

HOW TO EAT WELL

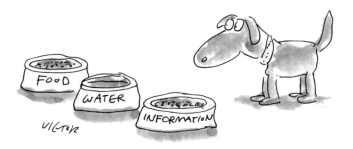

Boy, am I lucky! I live at Canyon Ranch and eat wonderful, healthy food every day, so thinking about nutrition is not something I ever have to do. You are going to have to work a little harder, but this chapter can help clear away some of the confusion that makes the basic act of nourishing yourself so complicated.

One problem people have eating well today is that they feel overwhelmed by all the often confusing, seemingly conflicting information about nutrition that floods the media: Eggs used to be "bad," then they were OK from a cholesterol point of view, but then they're bad again because of salmonella. Or are they? And what's the deal with high-fructose corn syrup, anyway? Our Canyon Ranch nutritionists stay busy sorting through the never-ending flow of new studies that so often appear to contradict previous studies.

You really don't need to pay attention to the babble. Here are a few of the simple, easy-to-remember rules that our nutritionists—who read all the research and actually understand it—give our guests. Follow even a few of them and you'll be well on your way to a healthier diet. You'll also have a much easier time navigating the junk- and fast-food-laden "toxic food environment" we all live in.

HOW TO STAY FOCUSED ON THE GOOD STUFF

DRINK PLENTY OF WATER EVERY DAY.

Life arose from the sea, and every process in your body requires water. And many factors, including exercise, dry air, a hot environment, travel and massages, increase your need to hydrate. It follows that one of the most important health habits you can cultivate is simply to drink water and other wholesome, clear, unsweetened fluids—such as herbal teas, tea and mineral water—throughout the day. (Eating plenty of fruit and vegetables also helps with hydration. These foods contain a great deal of water in combination with other nutrients that your body needs.) To make water more appealing, get a carbon filter or reverse osmosis filter for your faucet and keep a glass or stainless steel pitcher in the refrigerator. Add ice and lemon slices, cucumber slices or fresh spearmint, if you like, for great flavor.

Our nutritionists encourage our guests who use sports drinks to select ones that are free of ingredients such as high-fructose corn syrup and artificial coloring and flavoring. If you buy sports drinks, look for ones containing fewer ingredients. Or make your own sports drink at home: Orange juice with a dash of salt.

SPLURGE ON COLOR.

The brilliant colors of fruits, vegetables and legumes come from phytochemicals, a varied class of miracle nutrients that scientists are just beginning to appreciate fully. You don't need a degree in biochemistry to choose a variety of brilliantly colored, simply prepared plant foods every day.

CHOOSE FOODS AS CLOSE AS POSSIBLE TO THEIR NATURAL STATE.

Less processed is better than highly processed; simpler is better than complicated; whole is better than refined. Examples: Corn on the cob is better than tortilla chips; an apple is better than apple juice; broiled chicken is better than a chicken nugget. Processed foods are almost always higher in fat, sugar and sodium, and lower in fiber and other important nutrients than foods in a close-to-natural state.

FILL ¾ OF YOUR PLATE WITH PLANTS AND PROTEIN.

Most of your plate should be filled with quality protein and wholesomely prepared vegetables, fruits, whole grains and legumes. Just one quarter should be lean protein. Maintain this balance even when you snack and you'll be well on your way to an effortlessly excellent diet. Beverages from plants count too. Coffee, tea and herbal teas are wholesome plant products, and offer health benefits when enjoyed without added sweeteners and fats.

BE PICKY ABOUT FATS.

Extra-virgin olive oil, canola oil and the oils found in cold-water fish, seeds, nuts and avocados are the best fats for you. You absolutely require some fat as part of a healthy diet, but because all fats are calorie-dense, you need to watch the amount of fat and fatty foods you consume. So be particular about which fats you choose, and be sure they're fresh. (Store oils in the refrigerator and throw out any that develop an "off" smell or bitter flavor—they've begun to oxidize.)

WHAT TO AVOID

LIMIT WHITE FOODS
(EXCEPT FOR CAULIFLOWER, ONIONS AND GARLIC!).

Simple carbohydrates such as white flour, regular pasta, white rice and potatoes act almost like pure sugar on your blood-sugar level, raising it quickly and then letting it drop with a crash. Over time, this pattern can contribute to the development of insulin resistance and type 2 diabetes in people who are genetically predisposed to it (which is most of us!), and is associated with heart disease and other serious chronic illnesses. So do you have to say goodbye to starch forever? No. Just make a habit of selecting unrefined, whole-grain carbohydrates—the germ and fiber make a big difference to your body.

JUST SAY "NO" TO JUNK FOOD (INCLUDING SODA).

Junk food is expensive, fattening and terrible for you, and there's increasing evidence that it's actually addictive. Cut your consumption of nutrient-free highly processed foods gradually, if necessary, but do it.

AVOID FOODS THAT COME OUT OF LABORATORIES.

Artificial sweeteners and fats, preservatives,

genetically modified foods, high-fructose corn syrup—
Canyon Ranch nutritionists recommend that you avoid
all of them. The safest and best foods are those that our
bodies evolved over millions of years to use. We simply
do not know the long-term effects of molecules that our
bodies have never "seen" before.

HOW TO SHOP

SPEED-READ FOOD LABELS.

Look at the first three or four ingredients in the list
on the label, because by law ingredients are listed in order
of amount—the preponderant ones come first. If sugar,
salt or unhealthy fats are up at the top, put that package
back on the shelf. In addition, skim for polysyllables. If
you can't pronounce it, don't put it in your body.

EAT CLOSE TO HOME.

Look for locally grown food in health food stores and
farmers' markets. Food that's been shipped from another
hemisphere may not be as good for you—and certainly
isn't good for the environment. And try growing a few
things on your own. Gardening is a wonderfully satisfying
hobby. Even if you've never had a spade in your hand, a
basil or mint plant in a sunny window will brighten up
both your home and your table.

HOW TO HAVE A HAPPY (AND SANE) RELATIONSHIP WITH FOOD

BE ADVENTUROUS.

The more varied your diet, the better. Extend your reach, multiply your healthy choices and improve your nutrition by trying new fruits, vegetables, grains and legumes, exploring new ways of preparing familiar ones and by sampling various ethnic cuisines. It's a great big fascinating culinary world out there.

EXERCISE.

You'll be able to consume more delicious, nutrient-dense food—and, once in a while, that slice of chocolate cake—without putting on weight!

EMPOWER YOURSELF WITH KNOWLEDGE.

There are many reliable sources of up-to-the-minute food information online, and we list the best—ones our Canyon Ranch nutritionists and chefs rely on—at the back of this book.*

COOK.

When you cook, you're in complete control of what you consume. And cooking is fun, especially when you do it with friends or family. If you don't know how to cook,

*Page 113

you can take a class, watch how-to videos online, or get a friend to show you how to make some standards that you enjoy.

JUST EAT.

Create a regular eating habit throughout the day and never let yourself become ravenous. This is a key to moderate eating and healthy weight. Besides, it's only right to have a little respect and compassion for the needs of the body that carries you through life.

ABOVE ALL, REMEMBER THIS

DON'T PUNISH YOURSELF.

No matter how passionate you are about becoming healthier, don't try to make radical changes to the way you and your loved ones eat overnight. Eating is one of life's greatest and most personal pleasures, and we're all deeply attached to our established patterns and favorite foods. An exaggerated taste for sweetness or saltiness, for example, is created over time, and it will diminish with time as you gradually reduce the amount of sugar and salt you consume. Big, sudden changes are like extreme weight-loss diets—almost certainly unsustainable. Know that small improvements, sustained over months and years, add up to huge benefits.

chapter 5

HOW TO LOSE WEIGHT AND KEEP IT OFF

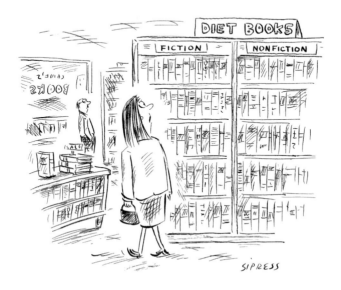

When I lecture on weight loss, I find that most people who want to maintain a healthy weight have been yo-yo dieters for lengthy periods. I know all about that. I've calculated that in my 30s and 40s I lost the same 20 to 30 pounds so many times that it added up to roughly 1,500 pounds. That's the better part of a ton! What a horrible way to live.

In those years, I was a "half gallon of ice cream a day" man. I knew I had a weight problem, and periodically I'd have a health scare, or just a moment of intense disgust with myself, and ask my doctor for a diet. Like most doctors in those days, he'd pull out the fad diet of the month and let me at it. So I've tried them all: grapefruit, high-protein, low-protein. If they'd had the lemonade and cayenne diet then, I'm sure I would've been on that too. The result: an incredible (and dangerous) yo-yo cycle, as I lost some weight on my latest unsustainable diet, then, in a few weeks or months, found myself right back where I started. Or, more likely than not, heavier than ever.

All these years later, there's still a ton of nonsense and, yes, even outright fiction out there about weight loss. The fads still rush in right around New Year's every year, just in time for us to resolve, one more time, that we'll lighten up for good. People reach for "extreme makeovers" or put aside logic to believe that this time, the Candy Diet or the Toast and Tuna Diet or the Eat All the Bacon You Want Diet endorsed by some skinny Hollywood star will do the trick.

Yet we know that fad diets don't work. Your diet is how you eat; it isn't something you "go on" when you wish to lose weight. The basics of losing weight and keeping it off are simple to understand, and they haven't changed much over the years—but that doesn't mean it's easy to stay on a healthy weight program in the midst of the craziness of everyday life.

Knowing what we know about obesity, though, it's crazy not to try. Obesity is associated with a galaxy of chronic health problems: diabetes, heart disease, orthopedic problems, many kinds of cancers, gastrointestinal disorders—you name it. If you want to keep those killers at bay, you need to maintain a reasonable weight. I guarantee that the healthy lifestyle that makes lasting weight loss possible will improve your level of wellness in many, many ways.

You don't have to deprive yourself of the pleasure of food to keep your weight within bounds—who would want a life like that? But you do have to be mindful and strategic. These healthy living rules will help with that, and make managing weight easier.

THE BEST THINGS YOU CAN DO
AWAY FROM THE TABLE

EXERCISE FOR 45 MINUTES TO AN HOUR,
FOUR DAYS A WEEK.

Ninety percent of the more than 10,000 weight-loss heroes on the National Weight Control Registry—people who have lost an average of almost 70 pounds and kept it off for at least five years—average an hour of exercise a day. That's what they've learned it takes for them to manage their weight, so that's what they do.

If you've got less to lose, you may see great results with a less rigorous regimen. But you will need to get regular exercise.

Exercise ramps up your metabolism because it tells your body to burn calories. You burn calories fast while you're actually exercising, of course, but you also continue to burn calories faster after a cardiovascular workout. Physically active people burn considerably more calories *at rest* than sedentary people do.

The very best type of exercise for turning up your metabolism? Interval training, where you work hard, then recover, work hard, then recover. But the important thing is not how you exercise, or what form of exercise you choose. It's that you do it.

In fact, one of the worst things about extra weight is that it makes it harder to exercise. (Obesity is a major risk factor, for example, for knee pain.) And that's bad because being sedentary is more dangerous than simply carrying excess weight. This is fact: Studies have shown that big people who are physically active are significantly healthier, on average, than thin people who get no exercise at all.

BUILD MUSCLE THROUGH STRENGTH TRAINING.

Muscle not only lets you move through the world and do what you want; having lots of muscle also gives you a tremendous weight-management advantage because muscle uses more energy than fat. That means that the more muscle you add, the more calories you can enjoy every day without putting on fat. Muscle is denser—more compact—than fat, so if you start weight-training, the number on the scale might go down more slowly than you'd like, but you'll look better and drop clothing sizes. (You'd probably be surprised at how much well-muscled people weigh.) And you'll be stronger and have better bones. Adding muscle to your frame is a total win-win!

STAY HYDRATED.

Many people think they're hungry when they're actually thirsty. Never let yourself get too dry. Drink water and other wholesome, clear liquids such as mineral water, tea and iced tea throughout the day.

GET ENOUGH SLEEP.

Lack of sleep depresses your mood, decreases your self-control, stimulates your appetite and increases insulin resistance.

THE BEST WAY TO APPROACH MEALS

SIT DOWN AND SLOW DOWN.

Take time to enjoy every meal and you'll be satisfied with less. The Slow Food movement, which perpetuates traditional styles of cooking and dining, is really on to something with this. People who eat slowly and mindfully, and who share leisurely meals with friends and family, are much less likely to be overweight than people who often gulp down food on the run.

START WITH A SALAD, CLEAR SOUP OR HOT BEVERAGE.

Take the edge off your hunger before the main course and you'll be less likely to eat too much of it.

WATCH PORTION SIZE.

Servings in many restaurants are ridiculously large. When you're brought a huge plateful of food, ask your server to package up some of it at the beginning of the meal. You'll have another meal for later, and you won't be tempted to keep mindlessly eating after you're full.

HOW TO STEER CLEAR OF COMMON PITFALLS

TAKE CARE OF YOUR METABOLISM.

Don't let yourself get too hungry. Eat balanced meals and snacks throughout the day.

TAKE CARE OF YOUR BLOOD SUGAR.

Limit sugary treats—and *never* consume them when your stomach is empty. (Have that piece of birthday cake as dessert after a good dinner—not at midnight.) Balance complex, wholesome carbs with lean protein and small amounts of healthy fats. And eat plenty of beans. They're full of fiber and protein and help keep blood sugar levels stable.

CHOOSE HEALTHY, HIGH-QUALITY FATS.

You need healthy fats as part of a balanced diet. We're more "liberal" now about the actual amount than our strict low-fat days—as long as they're healthy fats. That includes nuts, seeds, organic oils, nut butters, avocados, wild fish and organic grass-fed dairy and meats. And it's still important to watch your portion size.

DON'T EAT (OR DRINK) JUNK.

Most of what the processed food industry is trying to sell you is fattening, low in nutrients and high in sugar, salt, unhealthy fats and artificial ingredients. Don't bother finding out which burger is 50 calories fewer or a little lower in sodium than another. Just say no to all of it.

CONTINUE TO MONITOR YOURSELF ONCE YOU GET TO WHERE YOU WANT TO BE.

Give yourself a five-pound leeway so that you can indulge a little over the holidays or on vacation. But make that five-pound limit absolute. Yo-yo dieting is bad for your health, and take it from a veteran, absolutely no fun.

MIND-BODY SKILLS FOR HEALTHY EATING

Learn to comfort and nourish yourself through means other than food.

Do you need more sweetness in your life? More spiciness? Do you simply need more pleasure? Do you expend all your energy taking care of others and have none left for taking care of yourself? If the answer to any of these questions is yes, you may be trying to fulfill an emotional or spiritual need through eating. Exploring your inner world through journaling, meditation or counseling may help you achieve more control over the way you eat.

ACCEPT YOURSELF.

Your body may not be that of a model or a bodybuilder, but it's not your job to be on the cover of magazines, is it? You don't have to be perfect. You just have to be healthy.

chapter 6

WHY YOU NEED A GOOD NIGHT'S SLEEP— AND HOW TO GET IT

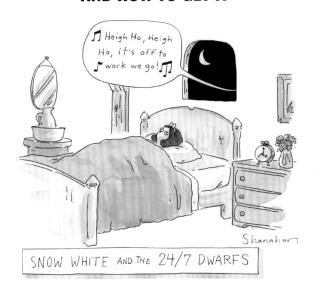

SNOW WHITE AND THE 24/7 DWARFS

I feel a bit hypocritical writing this chapter, because I am and always have been a terrible sleeper. I don't get many hours a night, but, by the measures below, I'm usually not sleep-deprived. However, our professionals at the Ranch see lots of people who are chronically sleep-deprived and who are in denial about it. Our physicians will tell you that trying to adapt to our 24/7 world is a very bad idea.

If you value your health and hope to live to a great age with maximum enjoyment, it's vital that you accept that your body's need for sleep is nonnegotiable. I'm still working on that.

HOW TO TELL IF YOU'RE SLEEP-DEPRIVED

DO YOU OFTEN:

- Fall asleep on airplanes?

- Need naps to make it through the day?

- Get sleepy in afternoon meetings?

- Fall asleep in front of the TV?

- Need caffeine to drive more than two hours?

If you answered yes to any of these questions, you're short on sleep.

YOU'RE SERIOUSLY SLEEP-DEPRIVED IF YOU:

- Fall asleep during church, class or meetings

- Fall asleep in waiting rooms

- Doze off during conversations

If you do any of the above, seek help from a sleep clinic or sleep specialist—your level of sleep deprivation is actually dangerous.

GET EIGHT HOURS A NIGHT, UNLESS YOU NEED MORE.

Our need for adequate, restorative sleep is as absolute as our need for exercise: Human beings can adapt to many things, but we *cannot* and *do not* successfully adapt to a lack of either physical activity or sleep. It doesn't matter how tough you think you are or how productive you think you need to be—you need your sleep.

A few individuals, and I happen to be one of them, feel well and alert with less, but we're the exception. The great majority of people need about eight hours a night for optimal health and function. And yet, in our overstimulated, hyped-up, Type-A world, millions of people are going around with much less than that. The result? Errors, accidents, pain, obesity, mood disorders, impaired immunity, attention deficit disorder and hyperactivity, and preventable chronic disease—plus a whole lot of just plain feeling tired.

IF YOU SNORE, YOU MAY WANT TO SEE A DOCTOR.

This is important if your snoring is punctuated by periods of silence or sudden snorts. Sleep apnea— periodically not breathing while you're asleep—affects between five and ten percent of the population and is a potentially dangerous medical condition.

If twitchy leg movements or hot flashes are keeping you awake or waking you up, you may want to see a doctor.

People tend to think of sleep problems as something they just have to put up with. They are not normal, and there is help. Restless leg syndrome is not a joke, nor is it an invention of the drug companies—and it is usually treatable. Similarly, the hormonal changes of menopause are a major cause of insomnia in women. If you're having trouble sleeping for physical reasons, your doctor may be able to help.

TIPS FOR BETTER SLEEP

IMPROVE YOUR SLEEP HYGIENE.

If you have trouble falling asleep or staying asleep for reasons other than the ones listed above, there are many things you can do to improve your sleep hygiene.

- Get plenty of exercise early in the day and get outside for a while each day.

- Avoid caffeine after lunchtime.

- Eat dinner early.

- Don't have more than one alcoholic drink in the evening.

- Turn down the lights and do quiet things as evening advances.

- Turn off the television or computer at least an hour before bed—the light and visual stimulation encourage wakefulness.

- Take a warm bath scented with a calming essential oil such as lavender; add bath salts to relax tense muscles.

- Take a mild analgesic, if necessary, to quell minor aches and pains.

- Have a cup of non-stimulating herbal tea or warm milk.

- Keep your bedroom cool and dark and use it only for sleep and sex—never for work or watching TV or texting/e-mail checking on your phone.

- Go to bed and get up at the same time each day; don't take naps.

- Turn the clock on the nightstand away from you.

- Make sure that everyone in your household respects the importance of a good night's sleep.

LEARN SOME CONSCIOUS BREATHING TECHNIQUES.

Breathing patterns that you can easily learn from an instructional CD or podcast can be very relaxing and can help ease you into sleep.

IF YOU'RE WAKEFUL, GET UP.

It's normal to take 20 to 40 minutes to fall asleep. If sleep just doesn't come, though, don't toss and turn. Instead, go into another room and do something peaceful and, preferably, a little boring, with the lights low. Especially useful is listening to a not overly exciting audio book. It's often our interior monologue that keeps us awake, and an emotionally neutral stream of words running through the brain overrides the anxious babble. Listening is better than reading, by the way, because anything that stimulates the brain's visual centers tends to wake us up.

IF YOU'RE STILL HAVING TROUBLE SLEEPING, SEE YOUR DOCTOR.

The latest generation of sleep medications is much safer than the old narcotics. Sleep is a cornerstone of health—take your need for it seriously.

INTERMISSION:

ADVICE FROM
THE DARK SIDE

QUESTIONS YOU MIGHT ASK AND
ANSWERS YOU MIGHT PREFER

TO HELL WITH HEALTH

THE DEFINITIVE POCKET GUIDE TO

GETTING OLDER FASTER

SHORTCUTS TO AGING!

FEEL-BAD TIPS! HOKUM, HOOEY AND BULLHOCKEY!

IT ALL MAKES SENSE

[TILL YOU THINK ABOUT IT!]

Q: I've heard that cardiovascular exercise can prolong life? Is this true?

A: Your heart is only good for so many beats, and that's it. Don't waste them on exercise. This is only logical—everything wears out eventually. Speeding up the heart to live longer is like thinking you can extend the life of your car by driving faster. Want to live longer? Take a nap!

Q: Should I cut down on meat and eat more fruits and vegetables?

A: You must grasp logistical efficiency. What does a cow eat? Hay and corn. And what are those? Vegetables. So steak is nothing more than an efficient way of delivering vegetables to your system. Need grain? Eat chicken. Beef is a good source of field grass (a leafy green vegetable). And a pork chop can give you 100 percent of the recommended daily servings of vegetables.

Q: How can I calculate my body/fat ratio?

A: Well, if you have a body and you have fat, your ratio is one. If you have two bodies, your ratio is two, and so on.

Q: What about smoking? Everyone tells me I should quit.

A: Look how many attractive people smoke! Movie stars, models, the Marlboro Man, Joe Camel. Would they smoke if it was bad for them?! Besides, smoking is relaxing.

Q: Should I reduce my alcohol intake?

A: No, not at all. Wine is made from fruit. Brandy is distilled wine, which means that they take some of the water out of the fruity bit so you get even more of the goodness that way. Beer and vodka are made from grain. Bottoms up!

Q: What are the advantages of participating in a regular exercise program?

A: Can't think of a single one. This is simple common sense: No pain . . . good!

Q: I've heard that swimming will improve my figure.

A: Explain whales.

Q: Aren't fried foods bad for you?

A: You're not listening! These days, foods are fried in vegetable oil. In fact they are permeated by it. How could getting more vegetables be bad for you?!?

Q: Will sit-ups help prevent me from getting a little soft around the middle?

A: Definitely not! When you exercise a muscle, it gets bigger. You should be doing sit-ups only if you want a bigger stomach.

Q: Is getting in shape important for my lifestyle?

A: Hey! Round is a shape.

Q: I've heard that walking is really good exercise. What do you think?

A: Long walks are great, especially when they're taken by people who annoy me.

Let's hope that this has cleared up any misconceptions you may have had about diet and exercise. And remember: Life should not be a journey to the grave with the intention of arriving safely in an attractive and well-preserved body. Rather, the goal is to skid in sideways, Chardonnay in one hand and a doughnut in the other, body thoroughly used up, and screaming, "WOO-HOO, what a ride!"

And for those of you who watch what you eat, here's the final word on nutrition and health. It's a relief to know the truth after all those conflicting nutritional studies.

1. The Japanese eat very little fat and suffer fewer heart attacks than we do.

2. The Mexicans eat lots of fat and suffer fewer heart attacks than we do.

3. The Chinese drink very little red wine and suffer fewer heart attacks than we do.

4. The French drink lots of red wine and suffer fewer heart attacks than we do.

5. The Germans drink lots of beer and eat lots of fat and suffer fewer heart attacks than we do.

The inescapable conclusion:
Eat and drink what you like. Speaking English is apparently what kills you.

chapter **7**

HOW TO MANAGE STRESS AND MOOD

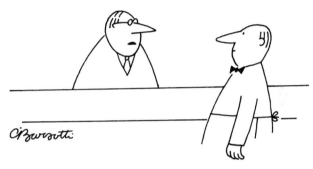

"A dash of hope, a dollop of optimism, a hint of courage—and gin—on the rocks."

Gin, on or off the rocks, is not the way to manage stress.

As a matter of fact, the only thing worse than the effects of chronic, uncontrolled stress is stress in combination with the sorts of things people often do to try to feel better, such as overeating, drinking too much, taking drugs and smoking.

In the years leading up to my "Aha! Moment," I was well acquainted not just with stress but also with the crazy ways a person can self-medicate it. Sugar was a big one for me. Cocktails. Taking my problems out on other people. I was on edge much of the time, and I count my lucky stars that my heart and blood vessels outlasted my regular spikes in blood pressure.

It's sobering to see how the body reacts when we don't have good ways of coping with the pressures of everyday life. The biochemical cascade that begins with the release of stress hormones, when triggered many times a day over years, can cause or worsen health problems. Research has linked chronically elevated stress to just about every known form of mental and physical impairment.

There are, however, highly effective ways to get a handle on your stress and manage your moods to be healthy. I've used a lot of them, and I can attest to the effectiveness of every technique on the list below. I'm by no means a laid-back guy, and there's plenty of stress in my life, but it's not killing me, or corroding my relationships or my pleasure in life. If rage, anxiety or frustration are problems for you, start here when you make a plan for steering yourself toward wellness.

GET SOME EXERCISE.

Yes, exercise makes everything better, and in the case of stress and mood, it's like first aid. This makes sense when you think about what stress chemicals are *for*—to help us cope physically in the face of a physical threat. Next time you're anxious or irritated, try taking a brisk walk. You'll feel better, guaranteed. And a good, regular exercise program will make your body and mind healthier and better regulated in general, so you can deal more effectively with life's problems.

MODIFY YOUR BODY'S REACTIONS TO STRESSORS.

Another approach to managing stress is to damp down the body's reactivity. Breathing techniques, visualizations, relaxation exercises and various forms of meditation are all useful and easy to learn. Hypnotherapy and biofeedback tools such as the emWave personal stress reliever from the Institute of HeartMath also work well. There's plenty of help out there.

ARRANGE YOUR LIFE TO BE LESS STRESSFUL.

Some stressors are unavoidable, of course, but many are our own doing. If stress is a problem for you, think about how you can change the things that add anxiety and frustration to your day. Allow more time to get places. Stop procrastinating or overscheduling. Shift your work hours to stay out of rush hour traffic. Avoid people who drive you nuts. No matter what your situation is, look clearly at yourself, and accept that you cannot change other people or the world. You can control only what you do.

PULL THE WAY YOU LIVE MORE CLOSELY INTO LINE WITH YOUR VALUES.

Many times, the grinding, serious stress in people's lives arises from a mismatch between their values—what they love and need—and the way they live. The man who loves human contact and conversation but is holed up alone in an office all day needs to change his life; so does the woman who values family above all else but works crazy hours. Sometimes the only cure for persistent, chronic stress is to make substantial changes—which is often difficult, and usually takes time. But if you're carrying a great deal of stress that's arising from a fundamental conflict between your values and your daily life, seriously explore how you can fix it. Seek professional help if you need assistance in working it through. Your health depends upon it.

LEARN TO SEE THINGS DIFFERENTLY.

Adjusting the way you see the world is the ultimate in stress relief. It's also the most difficult and transformative approach. It involves such profound change that it takes us deep into the realm of deliberately cultivating spirituality—which, by the way, has been shown to have significant health benefits.

Here's a story told by a member of our spirituality staff that illustrates what I mean by adjusting the way you see the world:

> *Once upon a time there was a great king whose best friend had been his pal since childhood. They did everything together. One of the remarkable and appealing things about the king's friend was his unshakable equanimity and positive outlook. No matter what happened, the king's friend would say in response, "This is good. God Almighty knows best."*
>
> *One day, the king and his friend were out hunting, and, as the friend handed the king his gun, he slipped, the gun fired, and the king's thumb was blown off. The friend leapt to stanch the flow of blood, and as he held a cloth over the wound, said, "This is good. God Almighty knows best." The king, in his pain and shock, flew into a rage. "You have gone too far! This cannot possibly be good! I am maimed and it is your fault!" He threw his friend into prison and left him there.*
>
> *Some months later, the king was out hunting by himself and wandered into a dangerous part*

of the forest, where he was captured by cannibals. They had him tied up and had set a big pot on the fire before they began to undress him. Pulling off his gloves, they discovered his missing thumb. They immediately let him go—the cannibals had an unbreakable taboo against eating imperfect creatures.

On his way back to the capital, the king reflected upon this course of events and began to feel intense remorse about how he'd treated his friend. He went straight to the prison. There, he ran to his friend's cell, threw open the door and hugged him, sobbing. Then he told him of all that had happened.

"This is good. God Almighty knows best," was his friend's fervent response.

"How can you say that?" said the king. "There was an accident, I lost my temper and threw you in prison where you've rotted for all this time, and for what? For trusting in God's goodness. And moreover, you were absolutely right—the accident with the gun just saved my life. It is so terribly wrong that you have been stuck in here!"

"Oh no," said his friend. "More than ever, I praise God. Because if I hadn't been in here, I would have been out in that forest with you!"

This story illustrates a truth that we often lose sight of: Our information about the world is never complete, and we truly do not know whether any single thing that happens is ultimately fortunate or not. You cannot see the future, so you might as well cultivate the attitude that everything that happens is for the best, because that assumption will reduce your stress. And, feeling less stress, you'll be clearer headed and better able to make the world a better place.

ABOVE ALL, DON'T LET YOURSELF BECOME STRESSED OUT OVER THINGS YOU CANNOT CONTROL.

Reinhold Niebuhr's Serenity Prayer has it right: *"God, grant me the serenity to accept the things I cannot change; courage to change the things I can; and wisdom to know the difference."* Very little in life, outside of our own bodies and minds, is within our control; the path to wisdom begins with recognizing this simple fact.

chapter **8**

HOW TO IMPROVE YOUR
EMOTIONAL RESILIENCE

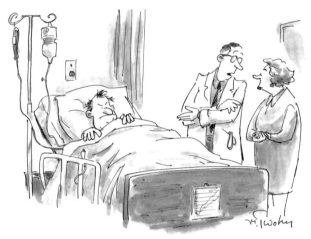

"He's one tough cookie. I've never seen anyone bounce back from an autopsy before."

Resilience is a hot topic these days, for good reason. Resilience, or stress-hardiness, is the difference between the POW who survives hellish conditions for years and somehow returns to everyday life a functioning human being, and the sad individual who's knocked down by life and never gets up. Individual temperament and life experience vary enormously, of course; that's what makes the similarities among people who bounce back so

8

telling. Psychologists now know a lot about the attitudes and coping mechanisms that keep people strong through adversity, and they've shown that they can be learned, practiced and mastered.

This is a subject that I find very interesting, because while I've always been optimistic and confident that I can think my way through any challenge, I am a very emotionally reactive individual. As long as I can *do* something, I'm great, and my emotional energy will carry me a long way. What I've found harder to deal with are those times and situations in which I have little or no control.

In difficult economic times, I've often found myself feeling sick with stress. What helped me was adopting this saying of the Buddha, and making it my mantra. Repeating it whenever I felt myself becoming upset and worried truly helped: *"The secret of health for both mind and body is not to mourn for the past, nor to worry about the future, but to live each day wisely and earnestly."*

Try it, and some of the other suggestions in this section. They can help you become a more resilient person.

ON THE PHYSICAL LEVEL

TAKE CARE OF YOUR BODY.

Good health, plenty of exercise and adequate sleep help create the internal climate for healthy thoughts and buoyant mood.

GET OUTSIDE EVERY DAY.

Spend time out in the fresh air. It's good just to be reminded that the natural world is there and that it hums along nicely without your having to control it. And there's nothing for lifting the spirits like seeing the sun shining.

EXERCISE.

Exercise is a fantastic stress reliever, and being physically strong makes you feel stronger emotionally. In addition, when you're getting regular exercise, you have one less thing to feel guilty and uneasy about.

ON THE MENTAL LEVEL

LAUGH.

I've put cartoons in this book for a reason: The benefits of a laughter-filled life are enormous. A person who sees humor in the absurdity of the world, and who is ready to laugh at his or her own reactivity and mistakes, has a way to reroute anger and reframe fear. When you take things lightly, you build your own escape hatch from stress. Ranch experts suggest that you laugh hard at least once a day—make an effort to regularly seek out the people and things that tickle your funny bone.

USE REASON TO COMBAT FEAR.

Recognize that if you do not achieve some distance from the primitive emotional centers in the brain that are devoted to fear, you will go through life ruled by worry, panic and rage. To be resilient, you must learn to use the rational thinking and judging part of the brain to manage your emotional core. Do this by watching for pessimistic, repetitive thoughts and actively disputing them. Is it *really* all your (or someone else's) fault? Is *everything really* terrible? Do you know *for a fact* that nothing will ever change, or that disaster looms? Use the powers of your mind to keep the danger-obsessed animal in its place.

STEP AWAY FROM USELESS THOUGHTS.

My friend Dan Baker, Ph.D., a gifted psychologist and the author of *What Happy People Know*, has a handy mnemonic for identifying unhealthy thoughts: **VERB**.

- When you begin to feel you've been **V**ictimized, stop!
- When you begin to feel **E**ntitled to more, stop!
- When you begin to long for **R**escue, stop!
- When you begin to feel that someone else is to **B**lame, stop!

These are useless lines of thought that sap your power to shape your life.

ON THE SPIRITUAL LEVEL

COUNT YOUR BLESSINGS.

Yes, it's a cliché, but it's also a powerful strategy for decreasing stress and increasing happiness. When you feel down or upset, try to turn your attention to what you love and cherish—deliberately practice appreciation. Don't do this because you should, or because it might make you "a nicer person," but because it's an effective technique for becoming happier.

> *"The hardest arithmetic to master is that which enables us to count our blessings."*
>
> – *Eric Hoffer,* Reflections on the Human Condition

chapter **9**
HOW TO CULTIVATE YOUR SPIRITUALITY

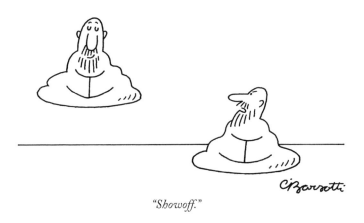

"Showoff."

I am not a conventionally spiritual person; at the same time, the spiritual aspect of life is very important to me, and has become increasingly so as I grow older. At one time, as a matter of fact, I jokingly offered to set up business as a guru when I finally achieved enlightenment. (My friends thought this was pretty hilarious.) The indelible image of me as Mukta "Aha!" Mel that graces the inside back flap of this book dates from that period.

Well, I'm still not enlightened, but I know a few things about the spirit and its role in making life better.

At Canyon Ranch we recognize that the most precious things in life are intangible. Things such as love, purpose, meaning and connection cannot be measured, but they are the very foundations of a resilient and motivated life.

These intangible qualities form the spiritual dimension. You may find your deepest connection to spirituality through formal religion, and, if so, good for you. But for me, as for many others, spirituality is not necessarily about religion, and certainly not about gurus on mountaintops. Spirituality is something universal. It's the way we make sense of life. It's what inspires us most deeply.

Our spirituality is guided by our experience of intuition, vitality and joy. The more you strengthen your spiritual self, the more your journey of wellness can thrive. Interestingly, the process works the other way too. Year after year, I see how our guests exercise their bodies hard, and in the process their spirits become softer and more receptive to the wonders and wisdom in the universe. There are many paths to the spirit. Here are just a few.

ACTIONS

BREATHE.

Learn some breathing techniques and use them: Any yoga or meditation teacher can show you how. Your breath is the bridge between mind and body, and mind-body practices the world over begin with conscious breathing. Counting, which is usually part of these techniques, serves a dual purpose: It helps regulate the rhythm of the breath while giving the busy, verbal left brain something to occupy it. This allows the intuitive, in-the-moment right brain to be heard.

TAKE TIME.

Make it a regular practice to do something that fills you with a sense of peace and connectedness. Whether it's prayer, meditation, a meditative physical practice such as yoga or qi gong, playing music, drawing, journaling or gardening—that's up to you. But do it.

MEDITATE.

Some people think that the point of meditation is to achieve stunning mystical revelation, but millions use it every day for very practical purposes—to cultivate positive emotions, lower blood pressure, improve clarity of perception and foster greater connection with others, for example. Research consistently shows that regular meditation makes people happier and healthier.

VISUALIZE.

Learn to use visualization, also known as guided imagery, to help you manage your stress and emotions. Deploying the imagination is a very effective way to shift your attention, and, in the process, convince the body—and the ancient parts of the brain that control it—that everything is OK. We have to learn to settle down if we want the spirit to expand.

Years ago, during a *really* stressful period—a big flood had sent the creek next to the Tucson property roaring up over its banks—I became so anxious that my neck froze completely. I could not turn my head. A psychologist rescued me, in part by teaching me to stop, breathe deeply and visualize warm, golden, luminous drops falling slowly on my forehead. I would try to see each drop fall, then feel it land on my head and gently roll down over my scalp. (This is a very ancient visualization, by the way.) I don't know what it was about that image that made it so relaxing, but it worked.

GET OUTDOORS.

Spending time in nature is both soothing and deeply renewing. We all ultimately come from nature, and we get back to our essential selves there. Whenever possible, enjoy the great natural daily events—sunrise and sunset, the first star emerging in twilight, the changing phases of the moon. There truly is nothing like a starry night sky for putting your preoccupations into perspective.

EXERCISE.

The ancient yogis invented yoga because they recognized that the body needed to be cared for before the spirit could blossom. As a Ranch guest wrote some years ago in a letter, *"At Canyon Ranch I've taken my body where it's never been, and my spirit has taken my soul to places it's always longed to be."* The body and the spirit soar together.

FEED YOUR APPETITE FOR BEAUTY.

Our senses connect us to reality, but while modern life furnishes a vast amount of stimulation, most of it is at the level of "noise" of one kind or another. You can nourish your spirit by seeking out and stopping to notice things that are deeply pleasing to your senses—whether it's music or forest sounds, beautiful photos of nature or great art, sensuous fabrics, lovely aromas, delightful sensations on the skin or delicious flavors. Beauty brings us into the moment, and the eternal present is where spirituality unfolds.

ATTITUDES

BE CURIOUS.

Instead of jumping to conclusions, ask questions. Everything we can do to come closer to the truth and step back from our automatic reactions helps us become more self-observant and more present in the moment. Part of being curious is listening—remember, you have one mouth but two ears.

FRAME YOUR DAY WITH THOUGHTFULNESS.

Make a practice of starting your day with clear intentions; end each day with gratitude. Do this faithfully and you'll find that you get more out of life.

GIVE OF YOURSELF.

Helping others who are in need will feed your spirit—and, of course, make the world a better place.

RULES OF THE ROAD

TRY TO TREAT ALL LIFE EXPERIENCES AS LESSONS.

Make a habit of stepping back. Ask yourself, "What can I learn from this painful situation?" "What is this annoying person teaching me?" Think of it as spiritual recycling: When you do this, nothing is wasted!

KNOW, LOVE AND FORGIVE YOURSELF.

The beginning of all kindness, all concern for others, is kindness to oneself. Practice forgiveness to free yourself of limiting thoughts and feelings.

FIND YOUR OWN WAY.

If ritual, be it secular or sacred, makes you feel connected to your life's meaning, engage in it regularly. Personally, I feel most spiritually alive when I'm with my family, or out walking, or exhorting guests to live right, or giving to a good cause. Every person's path is as individual as a thumbprint.

FINALLY, BE OPTIMISTIC.

In the words of Albert Einstein—who knew a thing or two: *"Learn from yesterday, live for today, hope for tomorrow."*

chapter **10**

YOU SHOULD KNOW ABOUT ENERGY HEALING

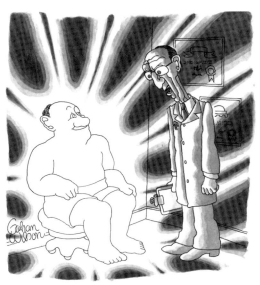

"You've been fooling around with alternative medicines, haven't you?"

From its earliest days, Canyon Ranch has been about helping people heal their bodies and spirits. I realized early on that massage and body workers had something to offer that went beyond soothing sore muscles, and year by year, we began to explore a wide array of therapies that balance and clear the flow of subtle energy through the body. (This energy is known as *qi*—pronounced *chi*—in China, as *prana* in India and by other names in other cultures.)

10

In some circles, the mention of something such as "subtle energy" may still seem "fringe-y" or unproven, but our integrative medicine experts have long recognized that many forms of hands-on energy healing are safe and effective. In fact, members of our staff have been at the forefront of research into the usefulness of energy healing in supporting health and complementing conventional Western medicine. Our guests, who often come to us stressed out and looking for relief, love these services.

So do I. I have used acupuncture to treat pain, reduced energy and high blood pressure, with excellent results. I am also a true devotee of Healing Touch, which I have relied upon greatly in times of stress and low energy, and when I was recovering from surgeries. It has been immensely helpful, and I recommend it to anyone—there are no contraindications for Healing Touch.

Enid and I can both attest to the healing power of various forms of massage. We've made it part of our daily lives for decades. Skilled body work offers relief for muscle stiffness, of course, but it has many other benefits, including stress relief, speeding toxins from the body and encouraging healing. And, frankly, massage feels wonderful. As we constantly remind our mostly Type-A guests, physical pleasure is a very good thing.

If you've not considered these forms of energy healing, I urge you to check into them. You may find the information below a little technical, but I'd like you to see some of the science behind what may look like fairly esoteric stuff. And if you're intrigued, I hope you'll experience acupuncture or Healing Touch—or simply get a massage from a skillful practitioner.

ENERGY HEALING BASICS

WE ARE ALL ENERGY BEINGS. THIS IS NOT POETRY; IT IS SCIENCE.

"In a few decades scientists have gone from a conviction that there is no such thing as energy fields in and around the human body ... to an absolute certainty that they exist."

–James Oshman, Ph.D.

Physicists tell us that matter *is* energy, and vice versa. Our bodies are made up of countless molecules that vibrate along with the energy fields that surround us, and all the complex systems of life are regulated by streams of chemical and electrical messages. The electrical impulses of the heart are measured by electrocardiogram; those of the brain by electroencephalogram. The heart's energy can affect the brain's energy and plays a fundamental role in emotion and health.

For optimal well-being, body, mind, emotions and spirit must all be healthy and balanced. Energy healing practices address healing at all these levels.

Energy therapies are very effective for inducing relaxation.

When the body relaxes, it heals. We do not wholly understand the mechanism through which energy therapies—which include acupuncture, Healing Touch, shiatsu, Reiki, Jin Shin Jyutsu, craniosacral therapy and Polarity—encourage the relaxation response, but it has been clearly shown that they do.

Energy therapies are not faith healing; they can, however, definitely support emotional and spiritual growth.

By inducing relaxation, creating balance and helping to unify body, mind, spirit and emotion, energy therapies can be very helpful to people who wish to explore the landscape within.

Acupuncture and Healing Touch are the energy healing modalities with the most scientific validation and the highest standards for practitioners.

ACUPUNCTURE BASICS

ACUPUNCTURE ADDRESSES THE FLOW OF SUBTLE ENERGY THROUGH THE BODY.

The practice is thousands of years old and is widely used in East Asia for anesthesia and pain relief, for preventive care and for the treatment of a great variety of conditions, including anxiety, digestive health and plantar fasciitis. Hundreds of millions of people rely on acupuncture and the other branches of traditional Chinese medicine (including herbal therapy, massage, qi gong and diet therapy) for health care.

Designing double-blind research on acupuncture is difficult because of the nature of the treatment, but in the U.S., acupuncture for certain conditions—including reducing cravings in people who are quitting smoking—is reimbursable by Medicare. Standards for licensing vary from state to state; national acupuncture organizations can provide referrals.

ACUPUNCTURE IS NOT PAINFUL.

The idea that it will hurt to be "stuck with needles" keeps some people from considering acupuncture. This is a misconception. The sterile needles used by qualified acupuncturists are much thinner than any needles used in traditional Western medicine: They are about the diameter of a human hair. Acupuncture may elicit a number of physical sensations, but it is not painful.

YOU NEED NOT "BELIEVE IN" ACUPUNCTURE TO BENEFIT FROM IT.

Acupuncture is now used by many veterinarians on animals with good effect.

HEALING TOUCH BASICS

HEALING TOUCH ADDRESSES THE BODY'S ENERGY FIELD AND THE ENERGY CENTERS KNOWN AS CHAKRAS.

Healing Touch is a gentle, nurturing, entirely noninvasive practice developed (and largely practiced) by nurses. It's safe for people of all ages and in any state of health. Healing Touch practitioners usually gently hold areas of the body, but they can also hold their hands an inch or two away from the patient. Practitioners certified by Healing Touch International have undergone a two-year continuing education training program and board certification.

HEALING TOUCH HAS BEEN THE SUBJECT OF DOZENS OF CLINICAL RESEARCH STUDIES.

In these studies, which include four funded by the National Institutes of Health, it has been shown to be effective in reducing anxiety and length of hospital stays in coronary bypass patients, among others. Healing Touch is being used in all areas of health care and in many clinical settings to address a wide range of issues, including relief of stress and pain, chronic illness, back and neck pain, sleep disturbances, pre- and post-surgical issues, fibromyalgia, wound healing and emotional issues, including depression and grief.

I'm told that different people respond to Healing Touch differently, and that the same person may have very different responses on different occasions. For myself, I can say that a Healing Touch session always leaves me with what I can describe only as a lightness of being. On one memorable occasion, I actually had an out-of-body experience while receiving Healing Touch: I floated up and looked down at my body lying on the table! I am not what you would call a "way out there" kind of guy, and this is hardly something I ever expected to experience. But I did.

chapter **11**
HOW TO STAY COGNITIVELY FIT

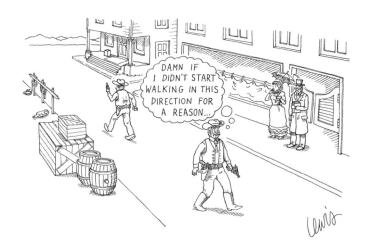

Nobody wants to forget where he's going or why.

Fortunately, there's a great deal you can do to protect your brain and reduce your chances of losing functionality with age. The news about brain health in the last few years is incredibly encouraging; we now know that the brain is much more plastic and resilient than we used to believe.

There's much you can—and should—do, especially if you've been pushing away anxiety about potential changes in your mind or memory.

11

TAKE CARE OF YOUR BRAIN

FIRST AND FOREMOST—LIVE A HEALTHY LIFESTYLE.

The most important way to ensure your mental acuity is to cherish and actively seek physical health throughout your life. The brain is part of the body, and *everything* you do to keep your body healthy benefits your brain. For example, the brain uses an enormous amount of oxygen all the time, so anything you do to enhance your cardiovascular health helps prevent dementia.

To put it another way: Processes that slowly compromise cognition later in life are associated with inflammation and elevated blood sugar; events that degrade it suddenly, such as stroke and aneurysm, result from high blood pressure and cardiovascular disease.

So, to increase your chances of having your full faculties until the end of life, live a healthy lifestyle. This is doubly important if you have a family history of senile dementia or Alzheimer's. Your genes need not be your fate!

EAT A DIET RICH IN ANTI-INFLAMMATORY FOODS AND SPICES.

Blueberries, oily fish, flaxseeds, cinnamon and turmeric are among the foods that have been shown to reduce inflammation throughout the body, and to support brain health. If you don't care for fish, look for fish oil, either as a liquid or in capsules; it's rich in brain-boosting omega-3 fatty acids. If you're a vegetarian, freshly ground flaxseed and flaxseed oil can supply omega-3 precursors. If you don't like turmeric (the spice that gives curries their bright orange color), flavorless capsules are available. Basically, you have no excuse *not* to optimally nourish your brain!

HAVE YOUR VITAMIN D LEVELS CHECKED.

Low levels of vitamin D are associated with a four-fold increase in risk for dementia, and undermine health in many other devastating ways. Vitamin D deficiency is both silent and extremely common—individuals use it very differently, so taking a multivitamin may not be enough. The wisest course is to have your doctor check your levels and then follow his or her recommendations.

EXERCISE REGULARLY, AND NEVER STOP DOING IT.

Using your muscles triggers the release of chemical messengers that stimulate the growth of brain cells and the connections between them. There's evidence that a program of regular exercise can even *reverse* brain aging to some extent. All forms of exercise are good, but the activities with the most concentrated cognitive benefit turn out to be those that combine movement, learning and fast decision-making: Ballroom dancing and table tennis are two great examples.

GET PLENTY OF SLEEP.

"As soon as you go to sleep, the elves come out and start fixing everything back up," Canyon Ranch professionals tell our guests. This is true for every aspect of health, but a good night's sleep is especially important for memory—during the night your brain is busy cataloging your experiences from the day for future retrieval. Studies show that people of all ages—from preschoolers to folks in their 90s—are significantly sharper when they're well rested. Most of us truly need at least eight hours a night, whether we realize it or not. If you skipped Chapter 6 because you "don't have sleep issues," go back and take a look now.

WEAR A HELMET WHEN APPROPRIATE.

Head injuries are associated with dementia, so be sure to use reasonable precautions in protecting yourself.

Always buckle your seatbelt and wear the appropriate safety equipment for all high-velocity activities and for all the vehicles you use, including bicycles. It's also vital to set a good example for your children and grandchildren, and to impress upon them the absolute necessity of wearing helmets when they're doing anything involving potential impact. Emergency room doctors see far too many people who own helmets but weren't wearing them when it counted.

AVOID CHEMICAL DAMAGE.

Avoid excessive use of alcohol and understand the medications that you take. Be sure to consult with your physician about drug interactions and contraindications whenever you start taking something new.

EXERCISE YOUR MIND

GET AN EDUCATION.

There's a striking negative correlation between education levels and dementia: The more years people spend in school, the less likely they are to lose brain power as they age. Brain cells create connections among themselves as they are used, so more schooling correlates to more connections. That means highly educated people tend to have more cognitive surplus, so even if they lose some cells to aging processes, they still have plenty to spare.

This seems to account for the fact that brain autopsies of some highly educated individuals who functioned well up to the time of their deaths have revealed physical signs of Alzheimer's disease. These folks apparently had enough cognitive surplus to take up the slack.

NEVER FUNCTIONALLY RETIRE.

If you do retire from your job, find activities that give your days shape, purpose and meaning, and that keep you interacting with others. Everyone needs a reason to get up in the morning.

LEARN THINGS.

Keep learning new skills and pursuing knowledge about whatever attracts you. Whether your interest lies in bird-watching, the history of World War II, the stock market—or all three—it doesn't matter, as far as your brain is concerned. Like every other system in the body, it just benefits from being *used*.

STAY SOCIAL.

There's an increasing body of research showing that social interaction keeps the mind sharp. People who stay connected and avoid boredom and loneliness are happier and, not surprisingly, live longer.

MONO-TASK

DO ONE THING AT A TIME.

One study after another has shown that multitasking and distraction are the enemies of peak performance. When you're driving, drive. (You're responsible for two tons of metal hurtling through space!) When you're talking on the phone, talk on the phone. When you're walking, walk. Just saying "no" to the manifold distractions of the modern world can help you do everything more easily and efficiently. It will also make you feel calmer and more centered, and that, in turn, improves attention, judgment and memory. This is not easy to do these days, so you may need to work at it.

Try this: Focus at various times throughout the day on which sense is dominant. Is your vision, hearing, or sense of touch, taste or smell most engaged at this moment? Mealtime is a great time to practice focusing your attention—the smells, textures and flavors of food can be a revelation when we let ourselves be totally present for the experience of eating. Another exercise to bring you to your senses: Sprawl on the floor and let music you love wash over you.

MANAGE YOUR STRESS AND ATTEND TO YOUR MOODS.

Stress, anxiety, grief and depression all strongly affect memory and the ability to concentrate. It's important to recognize that your brain simply won't function at its best during tough times and not to let that fact increase your distress. No one is at his or her sharpest during a life crisis: You won't be all there right after surgery, between jobs or while grieving, so try not to let worry about confusion and forgetfulness make you feel even worse. And do seek help if your emotional burden becomes too great. There are many caring professionals out there who are willing and able to provide assistance.

IF YOU'RE WORRIED ABOUT YOUR MENTAL FUNCTION, GET AN ASSESSMENT.

If you find yourself worrying about your memory and mental functioning, talk with your doctor about having a professional assessment done. Most of the people Canyon Ranch professionals assess actually turn out to be doing fine for their age and are very relieved to learn that. An expert can also give you personalized advice and lifestyle recommendations.

chapter **12**

HOW TO AGE WITH OPTIMAL FUNCTION

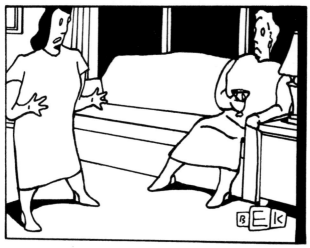

"Somehow, in all the confusion, I aged."

There is no way to avoid getting older. But you can definitely hedge your bets against premature aging and loss of independence. The secret, which should be no secret by now, is to live a healthy lifestyle. For me, knowing that it's possible to feel better at 89 than I did at 50 is the strongest possible motivation to keep living well.

We're learning a lot about living younger longer from research on that intriguing, rapidly growing segment

12

of the population, healthy centenarians. We now know that although your ultimate age is strongly influenced by genetics, how *well* you age is largely up to you. And the older you become, the truer this is. After all, modern medicine may save someone from an early death, but too often that simply prolongs the years of decrepitude. Ask yourself how you'd like to spend your last 25 years – full of vitality or dealing with chronic issues you might have prevented?

In particular, muscle loss (sarcopenia, to scientists) accelerates quickly with advancing age unless you work to stay strong. It is vital that you understand that the condition of the large muscles in the thighs and buttocks is one of the strongest determinants of independence and mobility in the later decades of life. Being able to get out of a chair or off of the toilet is something that we take for granted—until we can't do it anymore. As people get older, this one physical fact can become the difference between an active, happy life and a severely limited one.

It's easier to preserve health than to repair it. We can light the path for you, but only you can walk it. Every piece of advice in this book applies to successful aging, because living younger longer is the ultimate goal. Here's a summary of the key principles that contribute to a vibrant and enjoyable third act.

WORK.

Work hard at something you like—better yet, at something you love—throughout your life, and never functionally retire. Accomplishment feels good, and we all need to know that we're useful. Work is also invaluable for the way it keeps you in contact with other people and with the wider world. Isolation is the enemy—avoid it at all costs!

PLAY.

An active body and lively spirit are vital. Young animals and humans play all the time, and nothing keeps us young as much as doing things that are simply fun. Rediscover activities that have given you pleasure in the past and seek out new enjoyments. Brush up on your bowling skills, go out dancing, do puzzles, bake bread, play cards with friends, throw the ball around with the grandchildren or take them to a movie. Eat out with people you like. See the world.

EXERCISE.

"If we could put exercise in a pill, it would be the first anti-aging medication." My late friend Robert Butler, MD, the noted authority on aging, said this when he testified before the Senate Committee on Aging. There is no such pill and never will be—there are just the endless benefits of moving your body. So leave your aches and pains behind. Limber up. Work off your anxieties. Digest and sleep better. And even if you've never been active, start now, because age is no excuse. If you are physically active, you will, of course, have to modify what you do as the decades go by—an exercise professional can help with this. Don't let the fact that you can't do exactly what you used to ever become an excuse for doing nothing.

TAKE YOUR DOCTOR'S ADVICE.

Know your vital numbers, seek medical care when you need it, and follow your doctor's advice. Never neglect the basics of good health. Don't, however, let being conscious of your body become an excuse for thinking and talking about nothing but your aches and pains. That's a trap, and a terribly limiting way to live.

TAKE EXCELLENT CARE OF YOUR TEETH AND YOUR FEET.

This may sound odd, but both are vital to successful aging, and both can be trouble spots as people get older.

The mouth has been shown to be a source of bacteria and serious infection—proper oral hygiene and regular visits to the dentist are vital. Flexibility of the legs is important to healthy aging, and it starts with the flexibility of the feet. In addition, balance and equilibrium are of vital importance to long-term health—and that, too, begins at your feet. If you have any concerns, see a podiatrist.

EAT WELL.

Few centenarians have poor eating habits. Plenty of fresh fruit, vegetables, lean protein and fiber-rich grains and legumes nourish body and brain, keep disease at bay and slow the processes of aging. (And occasional treats make life worth living!) Most people in the Western world who die young suffer from either heart disease or cancer. A balanced diet emphasizing clean and healthy foods is critical in protecting you against both of them. And if you eat an optimal diet, you'll slow the processes of aging by providing necessary nutrients and preventing cellular wear and tear caused by oxidation and excessive blood sugar. For people who tolerate alcohol well, very moderate alcohol use appears to contribute to longevity and heart health.

JOIN.

Be an active, constructive part of something bigger than yourself—a church or temple, a company, a charitable organization, a club. The camaraderie, social support and sense of shared purpose are invaluable. What do you know, what can you do, that could help a worthy organization get something done?

STAY ALERT AND LIGHTHEARTED.

Explore, learn and keep laughing. An active mind and a forgiving, easily amused temperament are the norm among people who age exceptionally well. Read the paper, take classes, explore the Internet. Read deeply about subjects that interest you. And always open those funny emails.

AVOID RUTS.

A critical aspect of successful aging is staying adaptable. Try new things and do familiar things in a new way. Pushing your boundaries, regularly getting out of your comfort zone a little and changing things around will help you remain mentally acute and emotionally resilient. Travel. Try a beginning yoga class or do tai chi at the park, learn to paint or make pottery, join a hiking club, learn a language or keep a dream journal. Write your memoirs so your descendants can know you better.

MAINTAIN GOOD POSTURE.

Posture matters. And it matters even more as the years go by. People often ask me how I manage to stand straight—shoulders back and head up—at my age, and I tell them that I owe it partly to trying to be conscious of my posture, but mostly to the accrued benefits of more than 30 years of almost daily exercise. Avoiding a stoop and a shuffle as you get older requires that you maintain good flexibility all over—especially a flexible spine—and a strong core. ("Core" is shorthand for the musculature of the trunk, which includes many interconnected muscles within the abdomen, back and pelvis.) There is only one way to stay flexible and strong as the decades pass, and that's to work at it, with a will. If you're concerned about your posture or your gait, a physical therapist or exercise physiologist can show you exercises that will help you stand, sit and walk taller and with greater comfort. Still, as always, it's up to you to do the work.

KEEP UP APPEARANCES.

Dress fully as soon as you get up, treat yourself to regular trips to the salon or barber, and indulge in facials and new clothes as often as possible. Looking good keeps your spirits up and cheers those around you.

GIVE.

What can you give to others? To the world? To the future? One recent study showed that retirees who volunteered their time had half the risk of dying during a four-year period as their peers who didn't. Consciously combat the stereotype of the selfish, grumpy old person by practicing generosity every day with all your heart.

HAVE PURPOSE IN LIFE.

It doesn't matter whether your goal is big or small, and it doesn't really matter what it is, but studies show that people who feel a strong sense of purpose not only enjoy life more keenly than those who just drift along from one day to the next, but also live longer. If you want to enjoy life and find fulfillment, never stop setting goals.

LOVE.

Keep your heart open. Make and maintain social connections and treasure your close relationships. Stay married, foster your family ties and cultivate a circle of friends. Nurture and share your wisdom with the young. Enjoy pets. To paraphrase a song Barbra Streisand made famous, "People who need people are the healthiest people in the world."

I wish you health and love.

Afterword

There you have it. A condensed but complete guide to transforming your health at any age. You can will yourself to the starting line, and then get going—no matter what you've done before. If you need to start small, go right ahead, but start.

It all comes down to believing. Believing that you can be an active participant in creating your own good (or bad) health. And believing that your health, like your life, is not static but evolves on a continuum that you can influence. Investing in your health now is sure to yield benefits. Remember, you are the best doctor you will ever have. We all get stuck in our ruts—I was stuck in one for the first five decades of my life. But I got out of it. And you too can choose to put yourself in charge of the life you hope to lead. No, you can't cheat mortality by an act of will, but you can prevent, delay or eliminate many of the ill effects of an unhealthy lifestyle. The basics of living a healthy lifestyle are not negotiable: Get off the couch, put down your fork and your glass, and find some creative outlets to deflate your stress. It's not rocket science. Choose well, follow the smart advice in these pages, and before you know it, you'll feel the difference. Aim toward that healthy 100 mark and never look back.

Here's what I want you to take away: Don't do what I did for the first 50 years of my life. Do what I've done since.

Decide to live healthier. Only you can do it. I can tell you that carrying through on your decision will take commitment, self-discipline and a positive, can-do attitude, but that it will yield lifelong dividends, starting today: You'll perform better, look better and feel better about yourself. You'll enjoy better quality of life every day when you exercise regularly, eat a good diet and create balance in the way you live. The more you improve your level of health, the better your quality of life will become.

And the payoff becomes even more dramatic as the years go by. Every study that comes out validates the wisdom of investing that negligible three percent of your waking hours in regular exercise, with the biggest payoff coming late in the game. What we're talking about here is your quality of life from age 60 to 85, when so many physiological and biological changes take place in the body. Think about it—that's a whole quarter-century! The extent to which you are able to enjoy your later years is largely up to you.

So have fun and live life to the fullest. Have an "Aha! Moment" of your own. If a doubting, imperfect guy like me can do it, so can you.

Resources

The Canyon Ranch Guide to Living Younger Longer:
A Complete Program for Optimal Health
for Body, Mind, and Spirit
by the staff of Canyon Ranch with Len Sherman (2001)

Ultraprevention: The 6-Week Plan That Will
Make You Healthy for Life
by Mark Hyman, M.D. and Mark Liponis, M.D.

UltraLongevity: The Seven-Step Program for a Younger,
Healthier You
by Mark Liponis, M.D.

The Canyon Ranch Guide to Men's Health: A Doctor's
Prescription for Male Wellness
by Stephen C. Brewer, M.D.

The Everest Principle: How to Achieve the Summit
of Your Life
by Stephen C. Brewer, M.D. and Peggy Holt Wagner,
M.S., L.P.C.

Why Our Health Matters: A Vision of Medicine
That Can Transform Our Future
by Andrew Weil, M.D.

EXERCISE AND MOVEMENT

Healing Back Pain: The Mind-Body Connection
by John E. Sarno, M.D.

*Body, Mind and Sport: The Mind-Body Guide to Lifelong
Health, Fitness, and Your Personal Best*
by John Douillard

Prime for Life: Functional Fitness for Ageless Living
by Randy Raugh, M.P.T.

Treat Your Own Back
by Robin McKenzie

Treat Your Own Neck
by Robin McKenzie

Treat Your Own Shoulder
by Robin McKenzie

EATING WELL / HEALTHY WEIGHT LOSS

*The China Study: The Most Comprehensive Study of
Nutrition Ever Conducted and the Startling Implications
for Diet, Weight Loss and Long-Term Health*
by T. Colin Campbell, et al.

*Clean, Green, and Lean: Get Rid of the Toxins
That Make You Fat*
by Walter Crinnion

The Encyclopedia of Healing Foods
by Michael T. Murray, et al.

Natural Health, Natural Medicine
by Andrew Weil, M.D.

Prevent and Reverse Heart Disease: The Revolutionary,
Scientifically Proven, Nutrition-Based Cure
by Caldwell B. Esselstyn Jr., M.D.

The Food That Fits: A Guide to Mastering Your Food Style
by Lori Reamer, R.D.

The Volumetrics Eating Plan
by Barbara Rolls, Ph.D.

Women, Food and God: An Unexpected Path
to Almost Everything
by Geneen Roth

You on a Diet,
by Michael Roizen, M.D., and Mehmet Oz, M.D.

Canyon Ranch Nourish: Indulgently Healthy Cuisine
by Scott Uehlein and Canyon Ranch

The Hunter/Farmer Diet Solution
by Mark Liponis, M.D.

UP-TO-THE-MINUTE, ONLINE INFORMATION ABOUT FOOD, FOOD SAFETY AND NUTRITION

ANIMAL PRODUCTS:
Eat Wild—**eatwild.com**

FOOD ADDITIVES AND SAFETY:
Center for Science in the Public Interest —**cspinet.org**

FOOD SUPPLY AND POLICY:
Consumers Union—**consumersunion.org**
Institute for Agriculture and Trade Policy—**iatp.org**

LOCAL SOURCING:
Local Harvest—**localharvest.com**
Field to Plate—**fieldtoplate.com**

PRODUCE:
Environmental Working Group—**foodnews.org**

SEAFOOD SAFETY AND SUSTAINABILITY:
Monterey Bay Aquarium Seafood Watch—
montereybayaquarium.org/cr/seafoodwatch.aspx

SLEEP

The Harvard Medical School Guide to a Good Night's Sleep
by Lawrence Epstein, et al.

MANAGING STRESS AND MOOD / EMOTIONAL RESILIENCY / SPIRITUALITY

Breathing, with Mark Gerow (CD)
available from **lunarhythmsyoga.com**

The Energy Healing Experiments: Science Reveals Our Natural Ability to Heal
by Gary E. Schwartz, Ph.D.

Food & Mood: The Complete Guide to Eating Well and Feeling Your Best
by Elizabeth Somer, M.A., R.D.

Inspiration Deficit Disorder: The No-Pill Prescription to End High Stress, Low Energy, and Bad Habits
by Jonathan H. Ellerby, Ph.D.

The Mind-Body Solution: The Breakthrough Drug-Free Program for Lasting Relief from Depression
by Jeffrey Rossman, Ph.D.

Return to the Sacred: Ancient Pathways to Spiritual Awakening
by Jonathan H. Ellerby, Ph.D.

The Three Marriages: Reimagining Work, Self and Relationship
by David Whyte

What Happy People Know: How the New Science of Happiness Can Change Your Life for the Better
by Dan Baker, Ph.D.

Wherever You Go, There You Are
by Jon Kabat-Zinn, Ph.D.

COGNITIVE FITNESS

100 Simple Things You Can Do to Prevent Alzheimer's
by Jean Carper

The Brain That Changes Itself
by Norman Doidge, M.D.

*The Healthy Aging Brain: Sustaining Attachment
Attaining Wisdom,*
by Louis Cozolino

*How to Think like Leonardo da Vinci: Seven Steps to
Genius Every Day*
by Michael Gelb

*Spark: The Revolutionary New Science of Exercise
and the Brain*
by John J. Ratey, M.D.

30 Days to a Better Brain
by Richard Carmona, M.D., M.P.H., F.A.C.S.

OPTIMAL AGING

*The Blue Zones: Lessons for Living Longer From
the People Who've Lived the Longest*
by Dan Buettner

The Secrets of People Who Never Get Sick
by Gene Stone

*UltraLongevity: The Seven-Step Program
for a Younger, Healthier You*
by Mark Liponis, M.D.

Acknowledgments

Many thanks are owed to the Canyon Ranch professionals who have taught me so much over the years. I particularly appreciate the time and energy of the experts who reviewed the pertinent sections of the 2001 *Canyon Ranch Guide to Living Younger Longer* in preparation for this project.

Special thanks to Rich Carmona, Stephanie Ludwig, Jonathan Ellerby, Julie Haber, Sue Kagel, Ann Pardo, Lisa Powell, Steve Brewer, Mike Siemens, Param Dedhia and Gary E. Schwartz, all of whom contributed new material to this little book.

Thanks to the design team of Chris Sahlin and Teri Bingham, both of the Canyon Ranch Marketing Services department.

Thanks to Renée Downing and Bonnie Marson also of the Marketing Services department, who helped me with assembling the information here and assisted with the writing.

Many thanks to Morey Brown, who expertly shepherded this project from conception to publication.

Thanks also to Donna Frazier Glynn, our editor, and to Sheri Gordon, our copy editor

Cartoon Credits

Cartoons from *The New Yorker* are used by permission.